Dirty Talk

How To Engage In Erotic Communication And Elicit A Strong Desire In Your Partner Through The Use Of Provocative Phrases, Illustrated With Numerous Sensual Instances

Shane Charles

TABLE OF CONTENT

The Two Variants Of Erotic Communication

There are essentially two distinct categories of explicit communication to be aware of: soft-core dirty talk and hardcore dirty talk. Many individuals initiate their exploration into sexual communication through the use of mildly explicit language. The mild edition comprises language and expressions that lean towards a more affectionate tone. If you experience apprehension regarding engaging in explicit communication or are slightly uneasy about trying it, it is advisable to commence with more subtle expressions.

The beauty of indulging in provocative conversation lies in its versatility; it need not be entirely explicit. Engaging in provocative discourse involves both partners cultivating a level of comfort

that allows them to engage in playful and intimate interactions. Occasionally, even the most elementary matters possess a pleasing auditory and sensory appeal.

Consider exploring the realm of erotic language by incorporating certain expressions during intimate moments with your partner. Incorporate seductive communication into your prelude and observe the impact it has on your experience.

Illustrations of Mildly Explicit Verbal Communication
I greatly appreciate the sensation of your physique pressing against mine.
"Take me. I'm yours."
I greatly appreciate it when you bestow such affectionate kisses upon me.
I desire your presence within my being.
"You are so sexy."

Profuse obscenities and explicit language are more pronounced in hard-core explicit conversations. Profanity, informal language, derogatory remarks,

and hostility are more prevalent in the more intense rendition. With the utilization of explicit language, you have the ability to express yourself freely and engage in risqué conversation to any extent you desire. There truly exists infinite potential to depict detailed and explicit content. Due to this, individuals may occasionally become overly entangled and express derogatory remarks. Never hesitate to voice your concerns or express discomfort if you encounter any situations that make you feel uneasy or offended. Open communication is key. Moreover, exploring boundaries can be enjoyable and invigorating as long as one maintains a receptive mindset.

Examples of explicit and salacious verbal expression
Engage in intercourse with me using that phallus. Harder!"
I desire for you to engage in cunnilingus, thoroughly exploring and stimulating my genital region.
Do you derive pleasure from my fellatio?

I kindly request to be regarded as your intimate companion.

How to Customize Erotic Language for Enhancing Verbal Intimacy

Having an understanding of the distinction between mild and explicit forms of sexual communication can aid in determining one's personal boundaries. Please endeavor to avoid becoming excessively preoccupied with the disparities existing between the two. The manner in which something is communicated can often be more consequential than its actual content. Exclamations, expressions of discomfort, cries, breathy exhalations, faint utterances, soft spoken words, and menacing vocalizations have the potential to imbue any sentence with an unsavory connotation.

Various words and phrases may exhibit distinct auditory characteristics based on the modulation of your vocal tone. Attempt to modify the timbre of your voice in order to explore varying sexual

attitudes or roles. A shift in demeanor can determine whether one assumes a position of authority or subordination. Lower and huskier tones are generally perceived as indicative of dominance, whereas higher pitched and squeaky tones are commonly associated with submissiveness.

Assuming a certain demeanor or manner likewise enhances the exhilaration of engaging in explicit conversation. Expressing the desire for your presence within me possesses an inherent allure. Expressing the identical sentiment with a formal tone, adopting a submissive demeanor and alluding to the provocative nature of a nurse's behavior elevates the intensity of the scenario.

Conversational Indecencies Ought to Emanate Effortlessly

For dirty talk to be both enjoyable and stimulating, it is crucial for it to evoke a sense of authenticity and flow effortlessly. Verbal communication of a sensual nature ought to be a representation of one's state of arousal.

It serves as a means of conveying your preferences to your significant other. It is of utmost importance to exhibit spontaneity and articulate one's genuine feelings without an element of coercion.

Commence the discussion by addressing the present circumstances. Trust your bodily sensations and emotions to provide direction, thereby alleviating any sense of coercion or stress associated with engaging in provocative discourse. Providing a detailed and descriptive account is a simple task that effectively initiates action. Please attempt to phrase your response in the following manner:" "Kindly endeavor to express your thoughts in the subsequent way:" "I would appreciate it if you could articulate your sentiments using the following expressions:" "Would you be so kind as to formulate your ideas using the following phrases:" "Could you please try formulating your thoughts in the following fashion:" "May I request that you try expressing your viewpoint in the following manner:

I thoroughly enjoy the intensity with which you bestow your kisses upon me.

Your touch is quite soothing and comforting against my skin.

Please remove your trousers so that I may examine what is concealed therein.

I am becoming genuinely aroused by your presence.

It greatly arouses me when you passionately place your lips upon my neck in such a manner.

Go With the Flow

Occasionally, either you or your partner may prematurely exceed appropriate boundaries. In the event that such a situation arises and you happen to find yourself exhibiting laughter or light-hearted amusement, rest assured. It is entirely customary to exhibit laughter in instances where one experiences discomposure. Do make an effort to avoid causing your partner to feel insecure or foolish. Employ explicit language to reignite the intensity of the situation. "Employ the following phrases in order to regain composure after an ill-

advised conversation laced with impudence:

Could you please refrain from speaking and instead utilize your mouth for the purpose of kissing me?

Please be quiet and concentrate on providing oral stimulation to my breasts.

You are amusing me; perhaps you should engage in intercourse with me instead.

CHAPTER SEVEN
SOLID ADVICE FOR EFFECTIVELY ADDRESSING THE TOPIC OF SEXUALITY WITH YOUR CHILD

We are obligated to acknowledge the reality that certain matters will come to the attention of our children. Consequently, it is imperative for us to consistently and persistently provide assistance to them, effectively countering and moderating the myriad of perplexing stimuli they encounter within their sexualized environment, while aiding their comprehension of such stimuli.

By engaging in such efforts, we can anticipate making valuable additions to our child's reservoir of knowledge regarding sexuality. Please bear in mind that it is not necessary for our child's sexualized wall to be rigorous, perplexing, or detrimental in every circumstance.

As guardians, we contribute our own influences to our children's obstacles, and through effective and intelligent communication, these contributions can aid in the cultivation of a wholesome and favorable understanding of their sexuality, simultaneously mitigating the presence of undesirable barriers.

By elucidating our profound adoration for them and subsequently imparting precise information pertaining to sex and sexuality, establishing equitable and unwavering parameters for their sexual conduct, and offering counsel on comprehending the sexual stimuli they encounter, we contribute advantageous sexual notions to their sexualized framework and counteract the deleterious messages.

Presented herewith are five pivotal measures for you to undertake when commencing your endeavor to shield your child from exposure to plausible detrimental sexual stimuli.

• Acknowledge and comprehend the impact of these messages on your child.

• Take into account the approach employed in raising your children.

• Proactively engage your child in conversations about topics related to sexuality rather than waiting for them to initiate the discussion.

When feasible, leverage opportune circumstances for instructive purposes.

• Maintain awareness of your child's circumstances and exercise close vigilance over their activities and environment.

Let us carefully examine each one.

Acknowledge and comprehend the impact of these messages on your child.

Firstly, it is imperative that you acknowledge and affirm that your child is being influenced by potentially perilous sexual motifs. My son, who is in

his tenth year, exhibits a certain innocence that has been acknowledged by numerous parents regarding their own children's understanding or exposure to matters of sex and sexuality. He possesses limited understanding of human sexuality and lacks any inclination to deepen his knowledge in this domain. I am uncertain about his understanding of sexuality.

May I inquire about your current place of residence, if I may? In my personal conviction, it is my belief that parents adopting such viewpoints are merely deferring the acknowledgment of a disheartening trend in which we fail to recognize and appreciate the intellectual capacities, thoughts, and knowledge of our children. A substantial amount of evidence now substantiates this assertion.

We all desire to hold the belief that our children do not exhibit the same negative behaviors as other children. Nevertheless, it is imperative that we reconsider our preconceived notions

regarding the sexual behavior of our children.

Dear parents, it is imperative that we acknowledge the reality: Our children possess a natural inclination towards their sexuality. They contemplate the subject of sex, they have been exposed to relevant information and visuals, and their surroundings present numerous factors that may ignite their curiosity about sexual matters.

The factor of their age will naturally play a role. On average, a child of ten possesses a greater breadth of knowledge compared to a child of seven, while a child of seven exhibits a higher level of understanding than a child of four or five.

By the time she commences her education in kindergarten, your endearing child of either four or five years old will have engaged in a diversity of intimate encounters. When individuals of the age of twenty-five are collectively assembled for a substantive period, a discernible range of conduct and aptitudes, alongside diverse levels of

sexual inquisitiveness, will become evident. They will demonstrate it, and your child will also do so.

The predominant range of behaviors will encompass inquisitiveness towards dissimilarities in the anatomy of females and males, commonly referred to as the traditional game of "playing doctor." Additionally, it may include engaging in role-play as boyfriend and girlfriend, simulated kissing, lighthearted discussions pertaining to topics such as private parts, casual observation of others' living spaces, and naturally, self-stimulation.

Nevertheless, as I alluded to earlier, we are currently witnessing revelations from five-year-old children that were previously unfamiliar to us. Although five-year-olds exhibit innocence and naivety regarding matters of a sexual nature, instances of sexualized behavior in this age group are regrettably prevalent.

Currently, we observe children of this particular age engaging in physical contact involving their genitalia,

expressing desires in explicit terms such as "I desire to engage in sexual activity with you," observing instances where they exert force and coercion to undress others, make physical contact, as well as being aware of instances where oral sex is practiced.

I will delve further into this topic at a later stage, although I would like to address it momentarily because, given your role as a parent of a young child, it is crucial for you to acknowledge the susceptibility to sexually transmitted infections at this particular age.

It is imperative to exercise caution and avoid being excessively trusting concerning the exposure of sexual messages to one's child. If such is indeed the case, you may likely remain unaware of the utmost importance that lies in fostering an environment where your child feels comfortable engaging in discussions pertaining to matters of a sexual nature with you. If you hold the conviction that your child is wholly blameless, you shall bear the consequences. Your child will be

exposed to sexual signals and behavior earlier than you may anticipate.

As per the recollection of his kindergarten teacher, the young child inquired about the relationship status of one of his female classmates upon learning that she had a boyfriend, curiously inquiring about their level of intimacy. The mother of the young child was understandably distressed. Although not inherently concerning, these observations do suggest the evolution and transformation that has taken place over the course of time.

What course of action should a parent adopt in response to their child's disruptive behavior? Danny displayed erratic conduct and it would be inappropriate for him to have made the statement, suggesting that corrective measures should be taken. Be prepared to provide a comprehensive explanation of the concept of human sexuality should she display curiosity in pursuing further discussion. Should she find your response satisfactory, set it aside for the time being.

Please cease postponing it.

Proactively approach the subject of sex with your child rather than waiting for them to initiate the conversation. It is possible that she may never inquire about such matters.

It is imperative for parents to possess a level of knowledge and understanding on sexual development that surpasses that of their child, ensuring readiness for discussions surrounding sex and sexuality. After perusing the contents of this book, your comprehension will be enhanced regarding the precise information and timing required for your child's educational development.

This book will additionally enhance your comprehension of parenting concerns and approaches concerning our responsibility as sexual educators.

We did not pursue an education with the primary goal of acquiring the skills necessary to excel as parents; nonetheless, it is unquestionably the most arduous undertaking we will encounter.

Maximize the utilization of educational opportunities

Be prepared to intervene and assist your child in comprehending when you and your child are engaged in television viewing, music listening, or encountering a billboard showcasing sexualized content. Feel free to seek clarification without hesitation.

Engage in a meaningful conversation with your child about your emotions concerning the sexual content. Kindly impart your thoughts, opinions, and ideals to your child, should you deem it advantageous for their growth and development.

I will provide further elaboration on these instructional scenarios at a later point. This represents the primary method by which we educate and provide guidance to our children regarding matters pertaining to human sexuality.

Currently, let us assume that it will be necessary for us to acquire the skill of identifying instructional scenarios. A significant number of us maintain the

belief that engaging in formal, structured conversations regarding sex and sexuality with our children is imperative.

I am personally in favor of providing them with such guidance, although we primarily impart sex and sexuality advice to our children in organic circumstances.

If you happen to observe your seven-year-old engaging in self-stimulatory behavior on the couch within the confines of the living room, it would be appropriate to address the situation by gently stating, "Darling, I understand that the act of self-stimulation brings a sense of pleasure. However, as we have discussed previously, this is considered a private conduct, and I would greatly appreciate it if you refrained from engaging in it within my line of sight."

You are permitted to engage in such activities within the confines of your personal living space. Moreover, it is important to express your personal viewpoint on this matter, wherein you may either endorse or discourage such

behavior, according to your own discretion. However, it is essential to establish contextual limits by associating it exclusively with bedroom conduct. In an alternative scenario, it is possible for you to find yourself escorting your daughter, who is eight years old, to school in an urban area, only to encounter an establishment catering to adult consumers that prominently showcases a strap-on dildo and a nude inflatable doll.

Your initial response is to quicken your pace with the intent of avoiding any conversation. How might one approach discussing adult-oriented toys and inflatable dolls with a young child? As a conscientious caregiver, you acknowledge the importance of acting responsibly and engaging in a dialogue with your child regarding her recent observation.

The utilization of the commonly employed parental tactic of non-response, which numerous individuals resort to, is not permissible. I have been informed of multiple instances where

parents eschew challenging circumstances with their children, in the optimism that they will eventually depart independently.

They do not merely vanish; instead, they resurface to torment you. It would be ill-advised to allow these photographs to be displayed on her sexualized wall and exert their influence on her in the absence of adult supervision. The intervenor then interjects, saying, "The assortment of items displayed in that shop window was rather exceptionally unique, wouldn't you agree?" Observe her response. I have reservations about the possibility of an eight-year-old perceiving the presence of the item in question, but I am confident that she would indeed take notice of it.

"Why does this establishment carry an unclothed figurine and an artificial phallus?" she ponders aloud. You may acknowledge that, despite its peculiarity, some adults indeed purchase counterfeit phalluses and unclothed mannequins. Such a notion may appear absurd, yet it

holds factual accuracy. Certain adults find it amusing and engage in it playfully. Conversely, adults regard them with an authenticity akin to reality. My parent and I find it to be absurd, although I do not believe it would cause harm if certain adults desire them.

There is no need for you to be apprehensive about the potential detrimental impact of disclosing this information to your eight-year-old.

First and foremost, it is improbable that any of it will capture her attention. Nonetheless, I would suggest that you make note of her presence during these occurrences. There is a possibility of her encountering them once more, potentially on multiple occasions, should she opt to attend the educational institution adjacent to the establishment. In the absence of a proper framework for integrating the information, she may engage in discussions with her peers regarding what she has observed, potentially leading to an uncontrollable escalation of the situation. Aid your child

in understanding the perplexing information.

It is crucial to ensure that you act promptly and furnish appropriate context for the observations made, as this will greatly increase the likelihood of her retaining and integrating your perspectives. This measure will assist her in precluding any future involvement in the adult industry.

Observe

It is imperative that you give diligent consideration to your child's experiences. Maintain vigilant observation over his life and surroundings. This principle is applicable to all facets of parental guidance, but holds particular significance with regards to matters pertaining to sex and sexuality.

It is imperative to have knowledge about the associates, companions, and guardians of your child. This is an aspect that eludes the attention of numerous parents. It would be advantageous for you to acquaint yourself with the values held by your child's acquaintances. This

will disclose their sexual preferences to you. It also offers several advantages across different dimensions.

Commence your practice sessions at this time, as it will be imperative to direct your attention towards his peer group during the age range of eleven to fourteen. This particular phase presents a crucial period for fostering peer group relationships. Please ensure that if you own a computer, you take measures to prevent unsupervised access to it by children aged ten, eleven, or twelve.

Ensure that your children refrain from accessing Facebook or any other platforms of social networking. It is anticipated that you will be subjected to examinations.

Your daughter may inquire, "For what reason, Mother?" Your acquaintances are welcome to visit. Moreover, I hold deep affection for you, and taking into account your youth, I believe this form of virtual engagement is not suitable. Additionally, you possess unique qualities and exceptional character that set you apart from your peers, and

abstaining from this activity will be highly beneficial for you.

Adopt a resolute approach, particularly in the case of young children. They will vehemently protest, express their discontent, and persistently voice their opposition if you reject their request, however, that is regrettable. Inform them that you will not permit them to utilize the Internet or partake in any social networking platform unless under your careful supervision. Parents with children aged thirteen, fourteen, and fifteen ought to adopt a similar approach, particularly in regards to their engagement with social media platforms.

Take note of the manner in which your children engage with one another. In the event that there is a three to four-year age difference between your children, exercise caution regarding the teachings and behaviors exhibited by the elder sibling towards the younger one. Do not harbor the belief that the elder sibling will abstain from corrupting or causing

harm to the younger solely based on their familial bond.

The child of one of my clients, who is eight years old, engages in inappropriate behavior by prodding and touching the genital area and buttocks of their five-year-old sibling. She entertained doubts regarding the advisability of granting them further permission to partake in bathing. I provided her with my advice, recommending against the practice of bathing siblings of varying ages together. Please inspect the evidence in case you have any doubts about my claim. Grant permission on the condition of vigilant monitoring. If you are unable to provide supervision, allow them to bathe autonomously. Please ensure that you have implemented parental controls in your child's room, if she has access to a television.

Please ascertain whether your child has managed to decipher the codes despite the implemented safeguards.

Our youngsters appear to always be one step ahead of us in the technological world. We must not assume anything

when it pertains to the well-being of our children. They possess an undeniable charm and remarkable qualities that warrant a certain level of trust.

It is imperative to consistently bear in mind that your child possesses the capacity to engage in behaviors that are not desirable to you.

Develop the skill of perceiving from a broader perspective by maintaining a receptive attitude towards your surroundings. I was recently presented with the question of whether I believed it to be advantageous for a mother of a fifth-grade student to engage in surveillance activities to closely monitor her child's activities. I promptly responded, 'Indubitably, it is necessary.' What certain individuals perceive as intrusiveness, I refer to as diligent supervision, and it constitutes a vital aspect of responsible parenting.

As your children exhibit their competence and accountability in handling their own matters, it is only natural for you to be inclined towards granting them increased autonomy. You

should be aware that you are the one in control, and you will be overseeing their activities for as long as you deem it appropriate.

In regard to matters of sexual challenges, this holds significant importance.

Consider your parenting style.

There is an extensive body of research available on parenting techniques, providing us with a comprehensive understanding of effective and ineffective approaches in this domain. Upon analyzing the statistical data, it becomes evident that there exist four distinct parenting styles:

The account provided by the boy exhibits slight variation. As he was the individual who employed the term, you are allowed to inquire of him, "Are you familiar with the concept of sex?"

If he asserts that it signifies kissing or if he lacks knowledge on the subject, you can append, "Allow me to elucidate the meaning."

Intimate relationships encompass more than mere acts of affection such as kisses

and embraces. This can exclusively be accomplished by individuals who are of legal age and share a deep affection for each other, akin to that of a maternal figure and paternal figure.

The mother and father retire to their shared bed and engage in affectionate embraces and kisses. I believe the young lad has reached his limit by now. He would likely shield his ears and utter a remark along the lines of, "Disgusting, that is," culminating the matter. Due to the lack of interest that five-year-olds typically display towards discussions about sex, it is imperative for this young individual to understand the profound influence his words may carry.

POTENTIAL PARENTING APPROACHES THAT WARRANT CONTEMPLATION

• Authoritarian parents implement strict guidelines (\\\"Comply or face consequences\\\") and often resort to disciplinary measures to regulate their children\\\'s conduct.

• Permissive parents seek to establish a friendly rapport with their children

while avoiding confrontations and conflicts.

• Authoritative parents strive to maintain equilibrium, establish clearly delineated parameters of acceptable behavior, promote open dialogue, and utilize positive reinforcement as a means to shape conduct. This exemplifies the type of parent one aspires to be.

I will not delve extensively into the topic of parenting styles, but rather, I will meticulously analyze the components of each style in relation to the significance of a parent's accessibility in matters concerning sexuality, centering predominantly on the authoritative approach.

It would be advantageous for you to familiarize yourself with the advantages of authoritative parenting and endeavor to implement this approach consistently.

Phone Sex

Regardless of whether cohabiting or engaged in a geographically separated partnership, one can employ technological means to enhance their intimate experiences, such as engaging in telephonic sexual activity. If you are currently disinclined to engage in alternative sexual activities with your partner or are seeking to explore novel experiences, engaging in phone sex could be a viable choice. Whilst the concept of engaging in telephonic intimacy may evoke fascination, the initial foray into this realm can be fraught with uncomfortable unease. Engaging in sexual activity in solitude, whether through physical interaction or self-stimulation, is notably more uncomplicated due to the absence of any external observers. Nevertheless, it requires a distinct form of courage to engage in the potential act of sexual self-stimulation, in the presence of another individual through a video communication platform, wherein they

may potentially bear witness to and hear such intimate activities.

One must refrain from being excessively self-aware and consciously open themselves to engaging with the auditory and visual stimuli emanating from the other party in order to fully immerse oneself in the realm of phone sex, thereby enhancing its potential for an exhilarating and gratifying sexual encounter.

Furthermore, it is crucial to partake in meaningful dialogue rather than engaging in a monologue. A hypnotic session does not align with the nature of phone sex. It is crucial to ensure the sharing of each partner's actions, thoughts, and emotions.

Sex on Call

Create a strategy: While embracing spontaneity can enhance intimate experiences, it is possible to inadvertently contact your partner during inconvenient moments. Kindly

select a mutually convenient date and time to mitigate this issue. Contacting your significant other when experiencing sexual desire whilst they are having a difficult day has the potential to negatively affect your emotional state. Additionally, in the event that your significant other tends to be more reserved, it would be prudent to preface a sensual phone conversation by priming their mindset beforehand.

Establish a positive demeanor: It is likely that any feelings of discomfort or unease prior to your call will diminish the desired mood. Prior to the commencement of the call, make necessary preparations to establish the desired mindset. One may engage in dancing, partake in the consumption of wine, indulge in the reading of romance or adult literature, or even choose to view brief adult content. Additionally, one can cultivate a sense of sensuality by reclining for a period of time and adorning oneself in provocative attire. Prior to initiating the telephone

conversation, you may consider engaging in self-soothing gestures, such as tenderly comforting yourself, selecting and listening to your preferred tranquil melodies, retrieving any utilized objects designed for enhancing sexual pleasure, and adjusting the lighting to create a more subdued ambiance.

Establish communication: In the context of engaging in explicit telephonic interactions, there is no definitive prescribed structure. Notwithstanding, once

When your associate is engaged in a phone conversation with you, it is advisable to adopt a gradual approach. As a prudent measure, it is recommended to engage in a discussion about various topics before gradually shifting the focus towards discussions of a sexual nature. Do not hesitate to emit vocal expressions, employing a subdued and mellifluous tone. Alternatively, deepened respiration may be employed provided that it occurs naturally. It is advised against deliberately attempting

to project an overtly seductive auditory demeanor.

Engage in a conversation regarding uncomplicated matters: Despite the mutual understanding of the call's nature being centered around sexual content, it is not obligatory to directly address it. Commence by initiating discussions on benign subjects that can smoothly transition into enticing sexual discourse as the conversation progresses. Subsequently, draw inspiration from subsequent lines to grasp the techniques employed in this regard.

Could you kindly inform me about the clothing you are currently wearing?

6. The climate here is quite invigorating. I long for your presence in this place.

7. This bed is excessively large for my individual needs.

8. I am absentmindedly twirling my hair as I recline on the side of the bed where you typically sleep.

9. I longed for your presence by my side.

Could you kindly inform me of your actions involving your hands?

11. In the event of my presence with you at this moment, kindly elucidate how you would have engaged with me.

Engage in indirect and suggestive discourse when the appropriate atmosphere arises. Due to their absence in a physical sense, it will be necessary for you to employ elaborate and vivid language in your verbal expressions of intimacy. Both of you possess the capacity to provide a detailed depiction of your actions, specifically elucidating the manner, location, and nature of your tactile interactions, as well as providing comprehensive insight into your physical appearance, the objects involved, and any other pertinent particulars. "You may express it, as an illustration:

• In our initial enactment, I shall employ the whip procured from an establishment for mature individuals.

Currently, I am manually stimulating my genitalia.

• My nipples become taut when I am touching my breasts.

I am currently engaging with my undergarments, which are in a precarious position of potentially sliding down.

I am experiencing intense nausea and perspiration.

• I thoroughly enjoy the pleasant and engaging quality of your voice.

I am becoming aroused and moist.

I am gently combing my fingers through my hair.

To the resonating expression of your sensuous utterance, I am stimulating myself.

Please discuss with your partner a specific recollection from a memorable intimate encounter, for instance, an activity or desire you wished to engage in with them or a desire you would have liked them to fulfill. For instance:

9. I would greatly appreciate the opportunity to embrace you warmly and experience the comforting sensation of your supple skin.

10. I would appreciate the opportunity to tenderly place kisses upon your neck, lips, and décolletage.

11. Do you remember the manner in which you apprehended me from the rear during our previous encounter? I implore you to engage in a similar act of intimacy with me at this moment.

12. I am engaging in self-stimulation while contemplating the pleasurable sensations elicited by your touch upon my person.

13. Experience the gentle warmth of my breath against the intimate

freedom to unleash your true self by relinquishing any inhibitions.

One could express this idea in a formal manner by stating:

My pulse quickens upon hearing the sound of your voice.

When you speak in such a manner, it provokes an intense desire within me to unleash profound frustration.

Could you kindly reiterate that? I derive great satisfaction from hearing such remarks.

• The sound of your lamentations is deeply perturbing me. • Your mournful cries are profoundly unsettling me. • Your anguished vocalizations are profoundly affecting me. • The resonance of your expressions of distress is permeating to the very depths of my being.

I am of the opinion that it would be appropriate for me to accompany you in that location.

When you refer to me as your daughter, it evokes a sense of sensuality within me.

Currently, I am inclined towards embracing you affectionately.

I am ecstatic to announce my presence.

If inclined, one may partake in mutual stimulation or engage in self-pleasuring while sharing intimate vocalizations with their partner. Nevertheless, this is completely discretionary. If it doesn't evoke a sense of propriety or suitability, it is permissible to omit it. Furthermore, it is imperative to bear in mind that engaging in telephone-based sexual interactions does not invariably culminate in achieving an orgasm. It is permissible if neither of you attains climax or if only one of you achieves it. The primary focus of phone sex does not revolve around achieving orgasm. Nevertheless, should you find yourself having reached your climax while your partner has not yet achieved the climax, it is imperative that you refrain from terminating or muting the call. Please

proceed with detailing your emotions, aspirations, and related matters.

Conclude the conversation: Either party has the autonomy to terminate the call at any given moment. It is imperative to conclude the call prior to attaining orgasm. Furthermore, it is important to note that reaching one's pinnacle does not necessarily imply that the call should be terminated. You are permitted to engage in a brief discourse via telephone for any desired duration.

Deliberate on the matter later: Subsequently, do not hesitate to engage in a conversation regarding the telephonic intimacy. You may also communicate with them via text to express the exceptional nature of the experience. Notify them of your anticipation for an enjoyable telephonic interaction, expressing admiration and appreciation either verbally or through written correspondence. Maintaining silence on the matter subsequently may give the impression of discomfort or remorse on your part.

Engaging in intimate activities remotely via a video conference.

One can engage in an intimate encounter "in person" via electronic means, through the utilization of diverse technologies such as FaceTime, Skype, Zoom, and similar platforms. The level of excitement may be intensified, especially among males, through the observation of your partner's behaviors, response to your words, and facial gestures.

Ensure that your internet connection is sufficiently robust for video conferencing, or alternatively, opt for telephonic intimacy to prevent potential irritation and disruptions that may undermine the ambiance.

Video conferencing platforms such as Skype enable individuals to engage in intimate interactions, harnessing the capabilities of technology. This form of sexual connection proves particularly advantageous for couples who experience geographical separation or when one partner's travel commitments

are frequent. It ensures that their sexual and emotional compatibility remains synchronized. Addressing the inherent clumsiness and vulnerability also reinforces the mutual trust and belief between partners. Methods for employing vulgar or inappropriate language on Skype:

Preparation

A significant proportion of sexual interactions on Skype do not take place in an organic manner. That provides you with a period to prepare and strategize the course of action for the session. Examples of this phenomenon include: hand-picking a playlist, meticulously illuminating a candle, carefully selecting a stimulating toy and/or lubricant (should one wish to engage in self-indulgence), or thoughtfully picking out one's preferred seductive attire.

Approach this occasion with the same seriousness as you would a formal date.

If you happen to have children or share living space with others, it is imperative to ensure that any potential disruptions are mitigated. Can you fathom the extent of awkwardness that would ensue? Ideally, you will have a few hours of solitude in the comfort of your own abode. You are satisfied as a result of the closed door and windows. Given the circumstances, it is necessary to approach the Skype date with the same level of seriousness and regard as a physical encounter. Dress in attire suitable for an intimate and alluring encounter. Direct your attention to your companion, therefore, put away the mobile phone, power off the television, and close any other application windows. Envision a scenario wherein you and your companion are the sole individuals in existence within the current timeframe.

Please provide a detailed account of your current activities and your desired pursuits. Your voice carries significant importance. The ultimate level of

intimacy is achieved when physical contact is no longer necessary for a meaningful connection with your partner. Furthermore, their ability to observe you proves to be advantageous. Nevertheless, an erotic ambiance truly stimulates the circulatory system. What particular assertions could you provide?

In this moment, I feel a strong desire to engage in various actions with you, as your appearance is incredibly enticing.

● Are you ready for me to transition into wearing my undergarments?

I am being rough with your hair while planting gentle kisses on the nape of your neck.

The woman stated, 'I perceive the sensation of your gentle caresses moving along my body.'

"I am envisioning that you are currently engaging in the act of licking me," she stated.

At this moment, I am contemplating the passionate intensity with which you engage in intimate activities with me.

Explicit dialogues conducted via Skype are aptly complemented by a variety of auditory elements such as moans and heavy breathing. They will promptly induce a state of heightened sensuality. If you are uncertain about what to express, you can consistently recite literature with explicit and sensual content without any reservation. If you possess a fondness for writing, you have the option of meticulously crafting your provocative discourse beforehand, thereby ensuring its authenticity and conveying to your partner its derivation from your own thoughts.

Sexting

Sexting refers to the act of transmitting sexually explicit messages through online platforms. As a result of technological advancements, individuals

are relieved from the discomfort associated with expressing these sentiments directly in person.

Conversely, individuals now have the ability to exchange explicit messages with each other. Prior to engaging in a romantic or intimate relationship with an individual, one may utilize the act of exchanging explicit messages, commonly known as sexting, as a means to gauge their level of open-mindedness. Conversely, techniques of engaging in sexually explicit messaging can vary, ranging from subtle to overt. Initiating a form of digital communication involving suggestive content, through the use of subtly crafted messages that have the potential to be misconstrued as expressions of romantic interest, is indeed a prudent approach. Subsequently, you are able to transmit messages of a seductive nature that elicit a positive response from the recipient. Ultimately, you have the capability to transmit provocative messages that

elicit a profound desire in them to engage in intimate activities with you.

How to enhance your self-perception when interacting with the female gender!

I would like you to fully comprehend and internalize a fundamental principle of the human mind, which elucidates the reason why certain individuals are capable of transforming their lives, while others remain stagnant, merely wishing and hoping for change. This principle pertains to the functioning of the human brain and mind, exerting significant influence over our capabilities and actions. "And now, I present to you:

Although your brain may be inclined to engage in something novel, typically the brain only executes actions that are familiar.

Essentially, my point here is that individuals tend to engage in habitual patterns of behavior. Individuals often have a tendency to operate within the

framework of their accustomed thought processes and emotional experiences.

Indeed, it is possible that they harbor a desire for alteration to some extent.

However, the fact remains that, when faced with a situation in the actual world, if one is accustomed to behaving, perceiving, and reasoning in a particular manner, simply harboring uncertain desires to become different will not bring about any actual change.

The essential component for achieving any substantial transformation is the practice of mental rehearsal. It is essential for you to acquire the skill of programming in a manner that is aligned with your preferred sensations, behaviors, cognitions, beliefs, and responses. This should be done through ample repetition so that your brain recognizes the new sensations, actions, thoughts, and beliefs as more potent, vivid, genuine, and familiar compared to your previous state.

I feel compelled to reiterate this point due to its significant importance. It is insufficient to merely acknowledge the desire to initiate a transformation. Merely contemplating altering the current circumstances falls woefully short in terms of adequacy. If you desire a transformation, particularly one that involves substantial divergence, it is imperative to conscientiously engage in vivid, mental rehearsing.

Currently, my intent is not to be the original commentator on the subject of mental rehearsal or its controversial counterpart, guided visualization. However, it must be mentioned that the majority of these methodologies, as they are commonly presented, are highly ineffective.

That is not due to the lack of concern from the individuals who educate or articulate about them. The reason behind this can be attributed to either the omission of crucial ingredients necessary for the recipe's success or the

inclusion of unnecessary components that are imprudent.

Allow me to provide you with some essential strategies to effectively utilize mental rehearsal, so that within a few brief weeks, you can fully recondition the subconscious layers of your mind to cultivate beliefs, attitudes, awareness, behaviors, and timing that will grant you an exceptionally charismatic confidence and influence with women.

The first essential factor: The significance of respiration. As I previously highlighted in the previous edition, respiration holds significant significance in effectuating any profound transformation.

We have the option to delve into various metaphysical explanations, but let us maintain a scientific standpoint for the time being, if possible. The empirical evidence suggests that in cases wherein individuals experience prolonged fear or anxiety, the limbic region of the brain responsible for regulating the

fight/flight response becomes increasingly susceptible to being activated by seemingly insignificant stimuli, akin to a car alarm being triggered by the mere presence of a cat.

If you fail to interrupt this excessive limbic response, any attempts you make to engage the other cognitive faculties of the brain will be undermined and disturbed, thereby requiring a significantly heightened exertion of self-control and internal conflict in order to bring about transformation.

We desire to accomplish tasks in the most efficient manner possible.

Therefore, the initial measure in conducting your mental rehearsal for empowerment with women shall be to allocate a period of ten minutes to engage in the aforementioned breathing exercises, as explained in the preceding post. If you are unwilling to allocate ten minutes of your time to achieve success with women, my suggestion would be to cease your efforts immediately, as there

are others who would benefit from the additional space on this planet.

Key Number 2: Comprehending and utilizing the two forms of visualization.

In any case, there exists a form of visualization that entails envisioning oneself within the images. It is akin to observing a personal film reel that captures one's own actions, experiences, and behaviors, providing a visual representation of oneself.

This image, which serves as a valuable tool for instilling motivation and establishing a comprehensive cognitive trajectory, is commonly referred to as disassociated. It entails observing oneself undergo an experience, while not actively participating in the scene, resulting in a limited or possibly negligible emotional connection to the feelings associated with being present in that situation.

The Influence of Connotative Symbolism

The second type of visualization pertains to a mode where one does not envision oneself within the images, but rather observes what one would actually perceive if physically present within the image, viewing the surroundings through one's own eyes. This phenomenon is widely known as associated imagery, and it is this type of imagery that holds the greatest utility in thoroughly practicing novel behaviors, responses, emotions, and thoughts.

The effective technique for mental rehearsal entails initially employing a dissociated series of images. Visualize yourself exhibiting the desired appearance, mannerisms, and behavior. Subsequently, transition to associated images by stepping into these mental representations and actively engaging in movement, speech, cognition, and emotions as you would during the actual situation.

Does this make sense?

Initially, observing the disconnected visuals of the trajectory you aspire to pursue serves to establish a reference point and course for your cognitive processes, enabling them to attain a comprehensive understanding.

Subsequently, perceiving the correlated visual elements and actively navigating the physical environment while simulating the corresponding bodily actions, vocalizing in a manner similar to natural conversation, and engaging in the actual behaviors that would be undertaken, effectively augments the specificity and intricacy of cognitive processing within the mind.

Prior to imparting this exercise to you, it is essential to bear in mind that the act of reprogramming your subconscious mind for achieving success in interpersonal relations with women is indeed a systematic process. It is essential to engage in repetition and dedicated practice in order for the novel

thoughts, attitudes, behaviors, and emotions to establish firm grounding.

Therefore, it is advisable to engage in this activity on a daily basis for a duration of 2 to 3 weeks before anticipating any noticeable outcomes, although some individuals may observe immediate effects.

OK then

Select a specific scenario or context in which you desire to enhance your authority and self-assurance with women.

Let us assume it pertains to the primary approach or approach in the context of walking.

The initial task I would request of you is to position yourself in a comfortable manner on the floor and invigorate your body through a series of breathing exercises (which I previously mentioned as crucial) or those found in reputable literature on yoga or meditation.

I kindly request that you proceed by envisioning a mental space wherein you hold the belief that anything can be accomplished.

"To accomplish this, initiate a process of mental reflection by counting in a reverse sequence:

Visualize the number 3. Observe it thrice, as in triple threes. Next, observe the numeral 2 and mentally project its image thrice, specifically as 2, 2, 2. Lastly, observe the first numeral, repeated thrice as exemplified by the sequence 1, 1, 1. Verbally articulate each number as you visualize it within your thoughts.

Now, stand up. Envision before you a circular shape situated upon the surface. Utilize your current bodily arm and perform the action of tracing the circle on the ground.

Direct your gaze towards the circular object and conceptualize it as a realm where unlimited possibilities can be

actualized. Where the potential of manifesting anything into reality exists. In a realm where limitless possibilities can be brought to fruition. Then step into it.

OK. Now, consider the scenario in which you aspire to exude increased confidence and influence in your interactions with women. Observe the depiction of your appearance when you exude such immense confidence. Visualize yourself engaging in the actions of acting, speaking, standing, moving, and experiencing emotions in accordance with your desired outcome.

This is the image that is disconnected from you.

Utilizing Your Corresponding Visual Aids

Now, proceed forward and envision yourself physically entering the image so that you are actively engaged in walking, breathing, and speaking from that location. Observe the true visual perception that you would actively witness if you were physically present. Experience the emotions that naturally arise within you.

Now, in order to enhance your confidence, I encourage you to transcend your own self-perception and assume the role of the woman with whom you are about to engage. Envision yourself observing yourself from her perspective, experiencing the same level of excitement she feels upon meeting you, and perceiving her internal dialogue exclaiming, "Wow...this gentleman is quite attractive."

Ultimately, disengage from her presence and rediscover your poised, formidable self while maintaining a sense of detachment. Psychologically instruct yourself that your inner self will manifest in a manner that possesses all

the requisite attributes, conduct, profound understanding, mindset, and impeccable timing essential for achieving absolute triumph in your interactions with women.

Principle #3 The Significance of Releasing It

Once you have completed your mental rehearsal and visualization for the day, it is imperative that you dismiss it from your mind and relinquish any hold it may have on you.

Frequently, we are instructed that in order to attain something we truly desire or effect a change within ourselves, we must consistently contemplate it, ensuring that our "objective" remains at the forefront of our thoughts.

Indeed, this excessive enthusiasm is an inherently valueless concept that serves as an impediment to personal progress.

It is imperative to ascertain the appropriate level of motivation required

to instigate transformation, entailing the discernment of when to contemporaneously disregard and release it from one's thoughts.

It can be likened to the process of baking cookies in an oven (once again, we are employing baking analogies; previously involving recipes, and now centering on cookies). If the dough is placed in the oven and the oven door is consistently opened every 30 seconds to determine if the cookies are cooked, they will not reach completion.

Indeed, this perpetual contemplation regarding one's progress or efficacy is simply an alternative manifestation of uncertainty. Indeed, it is evident that "hope" and "doubt" inherently possess identical qualities. They both involve uncertainty.

After completing the process of mental rehearsal, it is essential to relinquish attachment to it. Simply release it, remain calm and assured that it will be

readily accessible to you within the realm of reality.

Chapter 8. Reaching Euphoria and the Significance of Climax

This could potentially explain your engagement in the practice of tantric sexual activities. If that is the case, we shall proceed to comprehensively discuss the tantric orgasm. It entails a higher level of complexity than one might anticipate, and renders transformative outcomes in one's life.

What Is It?

The topic of orgasm is often regarded as taboo. Discussing or referencing sexual pleasure in the context of a meal or in the presence of family members is generally considered inappropriate, unless one resides in a household that fosters open and candid conversations about such matters. In more traditional settings, refraining from engaging in such discussions is either regarded as

socially unacceptable or simply not feasible. There are numerous aspects pertaining to orgasms that we tend to avoid discussing, primarily due to the taboo surrounding the topic. However, it is worth noting that orgasms can have an impact on various aspects of your wellbeing, such as your sexual health, mental health, and physical health.

There exists a considerable lack of awareness among individuals regarding the notion that not all forms of orgasms are equivalent, with one of the most potent experiences being the tantric orgasm. This is because it enables you to attain all your aspirations and mitigate the repercussions that arise in your life, thereby facilitating the realization of your true desires.

The tantric orgasm elevates your experience of climax and is commonly referred to as the whole-body orgasm.

Classifications of Orgasms

One can experience a non-sexual orgasm. An orgasm can be defined as the abrupt discharge of energy, which is not necessarily limited to sexual contexts. However, it should be acknowledged that there are orgasms that occur specifically during sexual intercourse.

A sexual climax refers to the culmination of sexual energy attained through the act of sexual intercourse. Nevertheless, it can also manifest itself at a varying degree.

Additionally, there exists the phenomenon known as the energy orgasm, characterized by the spontaneous discharge of accumulated energy. Are you aware that a seizure can be considered as a manifestation of energy release, similar to an orgasm? Yawning is too, so you can actually suddenly release a bunch of energy, and many times, this is a sudden, uncontrolled release.

Have you ever experienced a momentary surge of vitality followed by a

subsequent onset of fatigue shortly thereafter? This is the consequence of an orgasm, as it generally entails the abrupt discharge of energy followed by a sudden awareness.

One has the ability to regulate one's orgasms, as well as manage this abrupt surge of energy.

Tantric sex entails experiencing a euphoric state of heightened physical pleasure that permeates the entire body. It entails the rapid escalation, the eruption, and the subsequent discharge.

However, the tantric orgasm refers to an intense and profound orgasm that liberates the body, often resulting in increased sensitivity for individuals when they encounter it. It constitutes an immensely potent climax that is practically beyond one's control.

"The Peak of Pleasure in the Valley

The genital orgasm, often referred to as the valley orgasm, typically pertains to the experience of heightened arousal

focused on the genital region. This sensation is characterized by a distinct sensation of relishing pleasure, an abrupt crescendo, followed by a decline, ultimately returning to the baseline state. The experience entails a highly concentrated type of climax, which frequently, upon further intensification, bestows a full-body sensation, leaving you with a sense of both nourishment and exhaustion as you progress.

On the other hand, a full-body sensation typically manifests when the intensity of the orgasm is felt throughout the entire physical being. Frequently, individuals perceive this as a complete bodily outcry, yet it subsequently engenders the rapid dispersion of orgasmic sensations beyond the genital region, permeating the entirety of one's physical being.

The manifestation of this phenomenon is not solely attributed to audible screams and contorted movements, but rather, it is held within the sensation of the abrupt dissipation of energy, which

subsequently influences one's post-experience emotions.

Experiencing orgasm without ejaculation

The remarkable aspect of this phenomenon is that it can induce male orgasm devoid of ejaculation. It is in fact not overly challenging, and the primary explanation behind the ability of certain individuals to achieve this lies in the redirection of attention away from the genitalia towards the entire body, allowing for a heightened sensory experience. Consequently, the sensation of orgasm gradually permeates throughout the entire physique.

What are the reasons to strive for achieving this particular type of orgasm? We shall elucidate the various categories of both physiological and psychological advantages that ensue from experiencing a tantric climax.

The Advantages of Tantric Climaxes

Tantric orgasms diverge from conventional genitalia orgasms by providing an experience that extends beyond a mere physical climax. However, orgasms engender sensations of euphoria and pleasure, subsequently alleviating symptoms of depression, stress, and anxiety, while also serving to enhance the body's natural immune system response.

Furthermore, tantric orgasms afford the opportunity to expend a significant number of calories, induce relaxation, and alleviate tension throughout the body, extending beyond the realm of the genitalia. If you are experiencing a decline in the quality of your sleep, engaging in sexual activity can potentially assist in alleviating this issue. Additionally, it promotes enhanced blood flow throughout the brain and body, resulting in heightened mental acuity and improved cognitive clarity. Additionally, it mitigates pain, facilitates cell regeneration, and concomitantly

diminishes the effects of aging on the body.

Furthermore, orgasms elicit the release of oxytocin in the human body, thereby enhancing the experience of intimacy. A tantric climax centers around the release of this energy, fostering an enhanced sense of connection and deepening the bond between oneself and one's partner.

However, it encompasses more than mere physical advantages; it also serves to enhance your spiritual well-being. One notable aspect of an orgasm is that, subsequent to its occurrence, the body transitions into a heightened state of receptiveness, where all bodily regions begin to perceive the movement of energy. Unlike a traditional orgasm which solely affects the genitalia, a tantric orgasm extends this experience to encompass the entire body. It has the capacity to foster alignment in both the spiritual and physical realms, effectively enhancing the vibrational frequency of your physical and mental faculties. Consequently, it facilitates the

harmonious integration of various facets of your being. During the experience of orgasms, one's egoic consciousness diminishes, resulting in the attainment of a state characterized by boundless existence. Hence, sexual activities and the ensuing climaxes can be regarded as instruments of spirituality. Orgasms serve as a profound means by which to achieve enlightenment, thereby imbuing tantric sexual practices with immense potency. You experience heightened vulnerability and exhilaration, accompanying a significantly enhanced state of consciousness. This intimate endeavor possesses the potential, without question, to profoundly alter your being.

One can also achieve the manifestation of their desires in life through the experience of an orgasm. It encompasses not only procreation through sexual intercourse, but rather a wide array of possibilities. A lesser-known fact is that the tantric orgasm enables the practitioner to manifest their desires

and aspirations in life through the profound experience of climax. This enables you to direct all your attention to and fully immerse yourself in the moment of your orgasm. By focusing on this profound and intimate experience, you manifest all that you desire.

It should be noted that upon experiencing an orgasm, one releases the accumulative energy and subsequently projects the desired manifestations, thereby enabling the attainment of virtually anything one aims to achieve solely through this climax.

This idea appears somewhat unconventional, does it not? It is imperative to comprehend that this constitutes a procedural undertaking wherein the purpose is to actualize profound sensations and alleviate any detrimental ideations. It would be prudent to acknowledge the potency of this particular manifestation of climax.

What is the recommended frequency for experiencing a tantric orgasm?

That would be contingent upon the extent of your need. Certain individuals should consider the prevailing energy. Consider perceiving orgasms as a means of alleviating tension and attaining an elevated state, rather than utilizing them solely as a means of escape.

Although it is true that certain individuals do employ these means solely as a means to evade the challenging realities of our world, such endeavors will ultimately prove futile for your own well-being. That is not a responsibly managed application of the orgasm, but if pursued in a manner that promotes both personal well-being and possession, you will greatly enhance your overall condition.

Therefore, it is possible for certain individuals to experience a tantric orgasm on a weekly basis. Certain individuals, when it comes to the alignment of their spiritual energies,

may prioritize this practice above all others with great frequency. It is imperative to bear in mind that this requirement rests solely upon your own shoulders, as it pertains to your own desires in achieving a tantric orgasm, and ultimately, for your own self-advancement. Do not excessively concern yourself with the manner in which you accomplish the task, but rather direct your attention towards the process of executing it.

Exploring the Concept of Edging and Its Contributions to the Development of the Tantric Orgasm

One method to induce the tantric orgasm and corresponding experience is by purposefully prolonging the climax. This technique serves as a means to stimulate oneself into a heightened state of arousal, facilitating the achievement of more intense and vigorous orgasms, resulting in an enhanced sense of well-being and a more holistic physical experience.

Postponing or extending the duration of orgasms enables one to fully experience and appreciate their intensity, transcending the confines of pure sexual gratification and encompassing a broader realm of physical manifestation.

Engaging in gentle and deliberate stimulation is an effective method to achieve this, and it can be practiced either individually or with a partner. For males, it is commonly believed to induce exceedingly potent climaxes, although it also proves effective for females.

It involves reaching the stage of orgasm and subsequently halting the pleasurable sensations, repeating this sequence multiple times. It provides a profound sense of pleasure, facilitates the attainment of orgasm, and constitutes a significant component of tantric sexual practices.

An approach I often find effective is to initially practice the technique on your partner, and subsequently apply it to yourself. Your conveyance undertakes

this action, halts momentarily, and subsequently alters its course, alternating between stimulating one another to the point of climax, gradually descending, repeating this cycle, ultimately culminating after a moderate duration. It presents itself as a commendable method for individuals who frequently encounter swift climaxes to acquire a worthwhile encounter of this particular orgasmic sensation. It also serves as an effective means to invigorate the body, while providing ample entertainment.

This condition that one experiences does not solely arise from their reproductive organs. The concept underlying this is to experience the euphoric sensation within your physical being. This certainly evokes a distinct sensation. An orgasm can be described as a surge of vitality coursing through the body, and it is important to note that it does not necessarily culminate in ejaculation.

The essence of this concept is to experience it as a holistic sensation,

relinquishing the notion that it must be exclusively confined to the genital region. This evokes a profound and intensely pleasurable sensation within you. It does not necessarily imply the presence of discomfort or any disruptive sensation. The underlying concept is to perceive and harmonize with the intrinsic dynamics and interconnectedness of the various elements within your existence. It presents an opportunity for practitioners to cultivate subtlety in managing their energies, leading to a profound experience of the orgasmic state. It is an infusion of vitality, yet it does not necessarily need to manifest as an aggressive or overt phenomenon.

A nuanced and empathetic approach will facilitate the awakening of the ecstatic state within your physical being. It will facilitate an experience tailored to your specific desires within the realm of tantra, affording you the opportunity to achieve complete sensory relaxation.

Oftentimes, an effective approach in discerning one's preferences in regards to tantric orgasm is to explore and identify one's own bodily sensations, as well as the specific energies one wishes to channel and the various manifestations thereof. This can constitute a profound and enduring expedition, which one may not initially recognize as necessary to undertake in order to attain genuine comprehension. However, comprehending the intricate subtleties of one's own physicality will engender transformation, leading to the realization of a more profound and efficacious manifestation of pleasure, one that will undeniably be embraced. Tantric orgasms possess the potential to generate transformative shifts in one's life, providing a unique perspective on harnessing orgasmic energy. Gaining a profound comprehension of its nature is crucial in order to unlock the enduring impact and tremendous fulfillment this extraordinary sensation can bestow.

Chapter 9. Aspirations

Desire represents the initial stage within the sexual response cycle, which encompasses desire, followed by excitement, orgasm, and resolution. It encompasses both engaging in sexual fantasies and desiring to partake in sexual acts. The phenomenon of desire manifests prior to the experience of sexual gratification and before tumescence, which is the augmentation of blood circulation to the genital region.

Both males and females can encounter two sexual desire disorders. Hypoactive sexual desire disorder is characterized by a diminished inclination towards engaging in sexual activity. Individuals who intentionally evade engaging in sexual contact with a partner experience symptoms of sexual aversion disorder.

The experience of experiencing sexual longing is an inherent aspect of the human condition. It is an inherent trait of every individual in this world, and it is a right that even women are entitled to.

In light of this, their physiology possesses the capability to generate estrogens, which play a predominant role in stimulating sexual desires among women.

However, what constitutes sexual desire?

Sexual desire primarily encompasses the yearning for physical and emotional intimacy of a sexual nature. It can be characterized in numerous manners. Engaging in physical contact, ranging from more innocent acts such as holding hands to more intimate activities like sexual intercourse, is deemed desirable as long as it elicits sexual gratification. In more straightforward terms, it could be referred to as one's libido.

Based on multiple research findings, it has been observed that women tend to have a comparatively lower level of sexual desire or libido in comparison to men. This phenomenon arises from the fact that women tend to prioritize the emotional aspects associated with

engaging in sexual activities, rather than solely fixating on the physical act.

The clinical diagnosis of hypoactive sexual desire disorder (formerly known as inhibited sexual desire disorder) should be established when the clinician determines that the client experiences an insufficient or absent amount of sexual fantasies or lacks the inclination for engaging in sexual activity. This individual not only refrains from actively pursuing sexual encounters, but also declines to exploit easily accessible opportunities for such interactions. Given that a substantial percentage (approximately 20%) of the population fulfilling this criterion express contentment with this state, the diagnostic should be conferred solely if the diminished level of longing causes significant distress to the individual or affects their interpersonal bonds.

Certain individuals exhibiting diminished libido may exhibit specific

interest in a particular form of sexual activity or intimate with one partner while lacking interest in another, whereas others demonstrate a general disinterest in engaging in sexual expression. Hypoactive sexual desire disorder typically emerges in adulthood, subsequent to a phase of typical sexual desire. Certain medical professionals assert that a greater proportion of male individuals tend to express concerns regarding diminished sexual desire compared to any other sexual complication, and said decrease in desire frequently coexists with additional sexual issues.

The assessment of sexual desire is consistently made within the framework of a relationship, whereby an individual's level of desire may appear low solely in comparison to a partner's heightened libido. For instance, it is common for a woman's level of sexual desire to peak during her late thirties. If the husband happens to be of the same age, it is probable that his sexual desire

is experiencing a decline. As a result, she may express dissatisfaction regarding his relatively low level of enthusiasm even though his level of desire is within the normal range.

Individuals suffering from sexual aversion disorder engage in deliberate avoidance of any form of genital contact with a partner. They commonly experience distressing emotions such as anxiety, fear, or disgust when confronted with the prospect of engaging in such intimate physical contact. Certain individuals experiencing this disorder prefer to refrain solely from engaging in sexual activity involving the genitals, while finding pleasure in engaging in activities such as kissing and cuddling. Some individuals abstain from any actions that have even the slightest hint of being sexual in nature. In order to prevent engaging in sexual situations, individuals may consciously avoid forming partnerships altogether, disregard personal hygiene, or immerse themselves excessively in professional

or social endeavors, even including religious participation. Sexual aversion is a less prevalent phenomenon compared to hyposexual desire and exhibits a higher incidence amongst females as opposed to males.

Some individuals diagnosed with sexual aversion disorder may experience extreme distress and anxiety when exposed to sexual stimuli, and this condition often significantly affects the quality of their marital union.

Both sexual desire disorders can be delineated by analogous theoretical frameworks, yet the empirical investigations supporting these theories are frequently characterized by inadequate design and conflicting findings. Clinicians frequently highlight emotional issues within the relationship, such as anger or fear, and assert that the desire problem serves as evidence of a broader challenge in the relationship. Alternative: "Some argue that the underlying cause of the marital issues lies in the diminished level of desire,

thereby acknowledging the possibility that both arguments hold validity."

Another possible explanation alludes to experiences in the past, indicating potential causes such as parental influence in instilling highly negative attitudes towards sex, a restrictive religious upbringing, instances of sexual abuse, or cases of rape.

Sexual desire may be hindered by conditions such as depression, obsessive-compulsive disorder, or the use of various medications, including those prescribed for the treatment of hypertension or anxiety. If these factors are the exclusive cause for diminished levels of sexual interest, the clinician should refrain from diagnosing a sexual desire disorder.

Certain individuals experience decreased libido due to concerns regarding the potential repercussions of sexual engagements, such as unintended pregnancy, appearing imprudent, or acquiring sexually transmitted infections

(STIs). The prevalence of the AIDS epidemic has led to augmented sexual abstinence, particularly among female college students.

Identifying the origins of the disorder presents an opportunity to potentially mitigate the severity of the symptoms by altering the partner's conduct or modifying the prevailing circumstances. Certain sexual desire issues may arise from inadequate hygiene or persistent sexual demands from the spouse, both of which can be addressed through dedicated efforts and enhanced communication. Should the concerns regarding potential negative repercussions of engaging in sexual activity prove to be unwarranted, it may be advantageous to provide instruction regarding the probable outcomes of such interactions. In numerous instances, nonetheless, it becomes evident that therapy needs to be focused on unveiling the concealed underlying factors contributing to the disorder.

Cognitive behavior therapy, although it demonstrates satisfactory efficacy in addressing various sexual dysfunctions, has not yielded comparable outcomes when it comes to treating desire-related issues. A prevalent cognitive approach observed in individuals with desire disorders is to engage in contemplation of unfavorable circumstances and concerns whenever they encounter a sexual opportunity. Given that this approach typically alleviates concerns surrounding potential sexual encounters, it becomes reinforced and subsequently exceedingly challenging to eradicate. Additionally, through abstaining from engaging in sexual activity, individuals affected by these disorders have limited opportunities to acquire the understanding that they might find pleasure in sexual experiences.

When women experience a dearth of sexual inclinations

However, despite women's permissiveness when it comes to

matters pertaining to sexuality, their lack of inclination remains a substantial issue. Whenever women experience a deficiency in their sexual desires, significant levels of stress and frustration tend to manifest, ultimately giving rise to depressive symptoms and an excessive number of insecurities.

The Deficiency of Sexual Desires in Women

Per the expert opinion of medical professionals, the inclination of women towards engaging in sexual activities can be attributed to a range of factors. In a general sense, this could be attributed to either physiological variances or psychological challenges.

In many instances, a considerable number of females experience diminished sexual desires as a result of the restricted production of estrogens. Estrogens are primarily the hormones synthesized by the female human body, playing a fundamental role in the development and regulation of one's

sexual desires. Typically, this situation may arise as a result of the medications women consume, specifically oral contraceptives.

Additionally, there are diseases that can induce a diminishment in women's sexual desires. Some potential causes for this condition include anemia, diabetes, and hyperprolactinemia, as well as an overactive pituitary gland. Additionally, it should be noted that addictions can result in a decline in women's sexual desires. Substance misuse and alcohol addiction may indeed constitute significant factors contributing to the gradual decline of women's interest in their desires.

Regarding the psychological issues that result in a lack of sexual desire in women, it can be definitively stated that depression and stress are the primary catalysts. It is comprehensible that in instances of significant pressure and uneasiness, a woman's focal point is liable to shift towards resolving the predicament at hand rather than

attending to her sexual desires. Furthermore, one could argue that the loss of interest in sexual activity is a direct consequence of unsuccessful relationships. This element is specific to the individual with whom the woman engages in sexual activity. In instances where discord arises within the partnership, it is highly probable that intimate yearnings and engagements may become suppressed.

Psychological issues contributing to women's lack of desires can also incorporate their emotional histories. Women who have had a history of childhood sexual abuse or any traumatic experience that may elicit fear towards sexual activities are more prone to diminished sexual interest when compared to those without such experiences.

Psychological factors can also serve as a classification for the inhibiting influences that cause women to experience a lack of sexual desires. Cultural norms and traditional values

are potentially influential factors contributing to the suppression of women's desires.

Identity may also contribute to the disparity in women's sexual desires. Latent same-sex attraction can have a profound impact on an individual, particularly when they are in a relationship with a partner of the opposite gender.

The Remedy for Women

Essentially, the treatment for women experiencing a deficiency in sexual desires relies on identifying the underlying factors that impede such desires. There exist a multitude of modalities to overcome this sexual disorder. Should the cause stem from a physical aspect, the administration of medical treatments could be recommended. If there are underlying psychological issues, it is highly probable that therapeutic interventions would serve as an effective solution.

Regardless of the remedy, women who experience a lack of sexual desires will only rekindle their interest in sexual activities through active self-effort. As previously mentioned, human nature encompasses the presence of desires, thus it is advised that women refrain from underestimating or disregarding this fact. In the event of an issue, it should be promptly addressed. In a different scenario, existence would undergo irrevocable alteration.

How to Enhance Libido

Each individual aspires for a harmonious, affectionate, and exemplary union leading to a nurturing and ideal familial relationship. In order to realize this ultimate aspiration, individuals must be receptive to certain alterations and must acquire the ability to embrace. The subsequent points outlined herein offer valuable suggestions on how to augment sexual desire and reignite marital relationships.

Maintain a healthy lifestyle. The maintenance of optimal mental and physical well-being is pivotal to fostering a vibrant and enthusiastic experience during one's intimate moments. More precisely, the initiation of passionate intercourse between married partners is facilitated by enhanced cardiovascular fitness, increased muscular endurance, and improved flexibility.

Acquire the skills of experimentation, exploration, and playful exploration. At times, engaging in monotonous and repetitive sexual acts, including foreplay, has grown tiresome and lackluster, consequently diminishing the allure and enthusiasm towards intimacy. In surrendering oneself to one's partner, it allows for both parties to fully indulge in and maximize the pleasure derived from intimate connection. In addition, by endeavoring to explore and innovate within various sexual positions, acts, and related methodologies, you can also enhance sexual appetite and fulfillment

for both yourself and your sexual partner.

Exude a powerful and undeniable charm, radiating with confidence and beauty that transcends both the inner and outer self. When you have acquired the necessary attributes to exude sexual allure, you effortlessly charm your partner - an enticing strategy to initiate a dynamic engagement in the realm of intimacy. Exhibit courage, audacity, and allure in his perception. When such circumstances arise, he can certainly decline your advances despite your appealing appearance. Undeniably, your paramount objective should be the enhancement of your partner's sexual desire. By captivating or enticing the individual, you do in fact achieve success.

Get the proper motivation. Gain a thorough understanding of your objectives and aspirations. Subsequently, proceed to implement everything. If you do not attempt the task, you will never ascertain the

efficacy of your techniques and the value of your endeavors. Enhance one's sexual desire, maintain concentration, and initiate physical activity. Nonetheless, it is important to recognize that excessive sexual activity can be detrimental, just as a complete absence or inadequate engagement in sexual activities can have even more negative consequences.

Maintain a youthful, amorous, and motivated disposition. In order to foster motivation and excitement, it is imperative that you also serve as a source of inspiration to your partner. Primarily, it is crucial to reframe the concept of sexual activity as an expression rooted in genuine affection, deep emotional connection, and passionate devotion. The primary factor to enhance sexual desire is to maintain a fervent, considerate, and intimate demeanor as a partner in the context of the bedroom. Exclusive moments shared with your lifelong partner can often be the most cherished and intimate experiences.

Undoubtedly, it is imperative that you perform a personal evaluation today and commence efforts to augment your sexual drive. By utilizing this approach, you will effectively optimize your time and resources, thereby enhancing the enjoyment and excitement derived from your enhanced sexual experiences. In conclusion, the aforementioned recommendations regarding methods to enhance sexual desire have been provided to you, and it is simply a matter of implementing them. To all couples, I encourage the cultivation of a mutually gratifying and controlled approach to intimate relations. Enjoy and fully appreciate every experience!

Puberty

All of the aforementioned points, however, shall be expounded upon in significantly more intricate and comprehensive manner.
What are the anticipated physiological, sociological, and psychological

transformations associated with adolescence for both genders? It is essential for girls to acquire the knowledge necessary to anticipate the onset of their initial menstrual cycle. It is essential for males to possess knowledge regarding the physiological processes of ejaculation and nocturnal emissions.

Fertility typically commences in females with the onset of menstruation, while in males it initiates upon the production of seminal fluid. It is a biological observation that both males and females are capable of reproduction once they have attained sexual maturity.

Sexual behavior

Certain children demonstrate an intrinsic fascination towards matters concerning human sexuality, while others exhibit a lesser inclination towards such subject matter. Both are normal. Once adolescence commences, individuals gradually begin to contemplate the notion of engaging in

sexual activity as a potential desire in their future endeavors. By initiating discussions on the topic of sexuality with your child, you are effectively conveying to them that they can approach you with any inquiries or concerns they may have. Additional information pertaining to sexual intercourse and various other sexual behaviors.

Fundamental details regarding STIs (Sexually Transmitted Infections) as individuals may come across them – occasionally, one may acquire infections through sexual intercourse, yet there exist methods to enhance the safety of sexual activity.

Fundamental knowledge on contraception methods can be employed to avert pregnancy - there exist measures that can be undertaken to prevent conception.

Familiarity with their parents' sexual principles and convictions, including but not limited to sentiments about love,

courtship, birth control, and appropriate timing for engaging in sexual activity. As adolescence commences, individuals gradually experience an increased awareness of their own sexuality and begin to cultivate romantic sentiments towards their peers.

Upon the onset of puberty, it is not uncommon for individuals to experience same-sex fantasies and attractions, which do not necessarily serve as determinants of one's sexual orientation.

The portrayal of sexuality in pornography is heightened.
How to practice cyber vigilance and employ safe mobile phone usage.

This could potentially be your final opportunity to engage in meaningful conversations with your child before they become less amenable to your guidance. As they enter adolescence, their reliance on peer relationships for knowledge and insight is increasing.

This implies that it is crucial to ensure their awareness of their ability to approach you to discuss any matter, regardless of its nature.

Therefore, it is imperative to respond candidly to their inquiries and furnish them with comprehensive information. In the event that you are unfamiliar with the answer to their inquiry, endeavor to collaboratively seek out the solution. It is imperative to not merely relay the information, but rather express one's perspectives and principles, particularly in relation to subjects such as romance, courtship, sexual activity, and birth control.

You will be required to employ ingenuity and explore alternative approaches to initiate conversations with them (offering them a book, engaging in conversation while chauffeuring, discussing mutual observations while watching TV).

Additionally, you may support their development of decision-making, communication, and assertiveness abilities.

Adolescence and beyond...

If you have not yet initiated discussions about sexual education with your children at this point, it is advisable that you take action promptly. Commencing these conversations is always beneficial, even though it may present greater difficulties later on.

During adolescence, sexual education begins to delve into more intimate aspects. It encompasses a multitude of challenging subjects including dating, contraception, determining the right time for engaging in sexual activity, and acquiring the skills to refuse unwanted advances.
One significant advantage of engaging in early conversations with your children is that it equips them with the information necessary to make well-informed

choices regarding sexual matters. Additionally, you will foster a connection with them in which they feel comfortable discussing any topic, without exception.

The information imparted to one's child holds significant importance, however, the crucial aspect lies in engaging in discussions surrounding it. This is the essence that holds significance.
Additionally, please be reminded that initiating a conversation is a timeless possibility that should not be underestimated.

This era is replete with emotional and social transformations, and young females, in particular, may encounter challenges related to body image. I strongly advocate for parents to engage in regular communication with their children regarding their emotional state and any inquiries they may have. At this stage of development, it is repeatedly underscored that these bodily changes are within the realm of normalcy.

Another aspect to consider normalizing is engaging in safe sexual practices. According to research findings, it is imperative to initiate discussions regarding sexual choices and safer sex practices by the age of 11. Admittedly, as a maternal figure, this concept may appear disconcerting, nonetheless, it is vital owing to the fact that teenagers tend to make more informed decisions when they are aware of the associated risks. It is advisable to emphasize various forms of contraception and elucidate the fundamental mechanisms underlying their efficacy.

Given the enhanced level of online autonomy typically associated with this particular demographic, it is advisable to engage in regular discourse pertaining to cyber safety, whilst further reinforcing the preexisting guidelines and principles governing their digital conduct.

For instance, engage in open and honest conversation regarding the potential legal ramifications of individuals distributing or possessing nude or sexually explicit photographs of themselves or their acquaintances. They may face charges related to the production or dissemination of child pornography, regardless of the consent or approval from all parties involved.

Inquire of your child, "What are your thoughts on the concept of demonstrating respect on social media?" When notable incidents of sexting or online bullying receive media attention, employ them as catalysts to prompt your child to express their approach towards handling comparable circumstances. Ensure that your child possesses sufficient media regulations on all technological devices.

Porn proof your child. Pornography often diminishes human dignity as it portrays sexual acts devoid of affection, closeness, or emotional connection. The

majority of pornography available today incorporates elements of verbal and/or physical aggression directed towards women, thereby posing potential harm to children who are exposed to such images and videos.

It is disconcerting for parents to acknowledge, however, it is highly likely that if your child has online connectivity, they will inevitably encounter explicit content. From a statistical perspective, the majority of children encounter explicit content before reaching the age of eight. As such, it is imperative that prior to this initial exposure, parents ensure the presence of effective parental controls on electronic devices and undertake the responsibility of educating their child regarding explicit material.

Educate your child about the fact that, much like how certain adults consume alcohol which is unsuitable for children, some adults possess a preference for viewing photographs or videos featuring

unclothed individuals, which is also unsuitable for children.

Reexamine your conversations pertaining to diverse facets of puberty as they increasingly manifest in the experience of your child.
Educate your preadolescent about the fact that entering the teenage years does not necessitate engaging in sexual activity, and express your desire for them to exercise restraint and postpone any sexual involvement until they find themselves in a committed and affectionate, enduring partnership.

Ensure that your preadolescent exercises caution when utilizing the Internet, refraining from divulging personal details such as age and location in public forums, as well as refraining from sharing passwords with acquaintances. Enforce regulations that prohibit the sharing of explicit photographs.

Ensure that your residence is a secure environment conducive to open discussions and inquiries, as you continue to engage in dialogue on previously introduced subjects. Communicate your principles regarding love and sexuality to your child. Inquire extensively, such as by asking:

At what point in a person's life do you believe individuals are capable of experiencing romantic love?

Do you believe that individuals should be married in order to engage in sexual intercourse? If this is not the case, how ought they ascertain their preparedness?

What are your thoughts on the alterations that occur with sexual intercourse?

In your opinion, how do you perceive the disparities between love and sexual relationships in reality compared to their portrayal in cinematic productions?

What would be the paramount attribute you would prioritize in the pursuit of a

romantic companion? How about considering royalty as a potential life partner?

Do you envision a future in which you will engage in romantic relationships with individuals of both genders?

What is the appropriate age at which individuals should enter into marriage?

Have you ever considered the possibility of entering into a matrimonial union?

What criteria should one employ to make the decision of choosing a life partner?

What are your views on the factors contributing to the dissolution of marriages?

Do you believe that any of the students at school have engaged in sexual activity? What is your opinion on the matter?

Is it prevalent for students at your school to engage in romantic relationships?

Are you acquainted with individuals who identify as homosexual or transgender?

Are they subjected to differential treatment by anyone? What are your thoughts/opinions on the matter?

Do you opine that males and females possess comparable requirements in terms of sexual and relational desires?

What are your thoughts on the concept of engaging in a "friends with benefits" arrangement?

In the event that you develop an affinity for another individual, what would be the most appropriate approach to manifesting this sentiment?

In a scenario where an individual desires to engage in a sexual encounter with another person who is incapacitated due to excessive alcohol consumption to the extent that they are unable to provide clear consent, what course of action should be pursued?

What recourse exists if an individual initially consents to engaging in sexual activity, but subsequently retracts their consent upon commencing the act?

Your fundamental responsibilities have been fulfilled. Please continue speaking

and, above all, please continue actively listening.

Engaging in conversations with your children about sex and sexuality at an early stage proves to be beneficial when they transition into adolescence. If you have positioned yourself as receptive to discussing those subjects, it is likely that your children will feel more at ease approaching you to ask questions.

However, if you have refrained from discussing the topic of sexuality thus far, I would suggest engaging in a sincere conversation with your adolescent and expressing your intention to modify your approach. Merely the act of listening to such information brings solace to the majority of children.

Whilst it is advisable to limit the amount of lecturing, it is imperative to engage teenagers in open and honest discussions regarding the topic of birth control. In fact, it may be beneficial to provide condoms or facilitate a medical

appointment for the potential implementation of hormonal birth control measures.

Regularly engaging in conversations about consent is equally imperative in the context of intimate relationships. Deliberation should be given to assisting individuals in safeguarding themselves against the influence of coercion and dating violence. Accordingly, discussions concerning these topics ought to incorporate an exploration of the potential consequences associated with alcohol and substance use, considering their impact on rational decision-making.

Regular discussions regarding healthy relationships are essential. Should your child display reluctance in discussing personal matters, I suggest engaging them in conversation regarding "acquaintances from school" to encourage discussion. Additionally, you may consider sharing anecdotes pertaining to your past relationships.

Ultimately, in regard to adolescents, your objective is to bestow upon your offspring the ability to assess potential hazards and exercise prudent judgment.

Facilitating children's comprehension of their instinctive discernment, internal guidance, and advocating for their attentiveness to such aspects form a significant component of comprehensive sexual education. By engaging in conversations on appropriate subjects at the suitable developmental stages, you are effectively equipping your child to accomplish precisely that.

You may be fortunate enough for your tween to come directly to you with questions. It is probable that you will need to actively seize opportunities in order to initiate the conversations.

It is possible that you may encounter this experience whilst engaged in the act of listening to a widely renowned song pertaining to the dissolution of a

romantic partnership. Perhaps it is when you discern a glimmer in your adolescent's gaze upon encountering someone who arouses their interest.

Alternatively, it may occur when you come across a condom discreetly tucked away in a desk compartment. (However, it is desirable that you initiate the conversation earlier.) This could occur when you become aware that the subject will be addressed in health education, and you wish to ensure that your child continues to view you as a reliable source of information." As you embark upon the initial stage, subsequent conversations will progressively become more comfortable.

This is not a singular occurrence.

While we recognize the utmost significance of engaging in discussions regarding sex and sexuality, it would be disingenuous to portray them as inherently comfortable to initiate. Hence, I am penning this literary work in

order to alleviate the difficulties. Keep this in mind: This conversation should not be referred to as "The Talk."

This infers a singular occurrence, indicating that once it concludes, there will be no further proceedings. That imposes an excessive burden on the subject matter. The discussion surrounding sex and sexuality should be a continuous dialogue.

A relationship that gradually and smoothly develops, while consistently reinforcing your principles and beliefs about the importance of a healthy sexual dynamic.

It is imperative to ensure that young individuals acquire accurate information about sexuality along with the skills necessary to effectively navigate and make responsible choices relating to sexual activities.

According to research findings, parents who engage in open and transparent

discussions regarding sexuality with their children are more likely to exert a significant impact on their child's sexual behaviors as they develop.

Allow me to provide clarification: It is imperative to acknowledge that sexuality and sex are distinct entities. Sexuality encompasses a diverse array of matters, encompassing an appreciation for our physical selves and honoring others' autonomy over their own bodies. Healthy sexual expression is intricately connected to interpersonal connections.

However, sexual activity encompasses bodily interactions that, when engaged in with consideration and within appropriate circumstances, can serve as a delightful aspect of the human encounter. It is imperative for adolescents to acquire knowledge regarding both in order to embark on a path towards a healthy transition into adulthood.

Is There A Social Stigma Associated With The Concept Of Engaging In Explicit Language During Intimate Conversations?

A significant portion of the negative discourse surrounding sex stems from our collective discomfort in engaging in conversations about it. We experience a sense of discomfort and unease due to the fact that during our formative years, sexual activity was commonly described as the "dirty deed," and masturbation was viewed as "self abuse" by individuals lacking sufficient expertise in this domain.

Furthermore, one could argue that societal conventions regarding intimacy and the vocabulary employed to express our desires and needs often suggest that the higher power responsible for bestowing upon us our physical form designed the limbs and torso, while attributing the creation of the remaining parts, which afford us the greatest pleasure, to an unscrupulous entity.

Despite the ongoing progression towards more open discourse on sexuality, the persistence of antiquated notions on permissible use of explicit language continues to influence the discourse surrounding the utilization of intimate vocabulary. An illustration of the ongoing taboo surrounding sex and discussions pertaining to it can be seen in the fact that in order to locate a discourse on this subject, one would have to input phrases such as "inappropriate language" or "discourse on sexual matters" into a search engine.

I continue to harbor a fondness for the term "dirty talk" as I have, in essence, reassigned its meaning to convey a sense of positivity. Furthermore, I am drawn to the thrill of challenging societal norms and the exhilaration of exploring the sensual realm.

Thus, we propose a redefinition of erotic communication as an affirmative and highly sensual form of expression.

◆◆◆

How to Cultivate Seductive Conversation and Enliven Playful Verbal Exchange

Dirty talk is:

expressing your desires and requirements.

granting oneself the authorization to verbalize one's sensual reverie.

Exploring the triggers that arouse your partner and amplify their exhilaration.

Pursuing the diverse experiences that add excitement to life, incorporating explicit verbal expressions known as "erotic discourse" brings significant variety to a close and personal connection.

Stimulating the most extensive erogenous zone available - your intellect and imaginative faculties.

◆◆◆

What are the reasons behind the enhancement of a relationship through the use of explicit language?

We transcend the boundaries of public discourse to engage in conversations reserved solely for our trusted confidants and companions.

We grant ourselves the liberty to express our desires, even if they are deemed inappropriate or excessively mature for public discourse.

Previously stigmatized subjects have the potential to be highly alluring.

Confidential conversations serve as a personal means of communication exclusively shared between you and your romantic partner.

You will experience immense satisfaction in kindling and maintaining fervent affection with your partner.

It fosters a deeper connection by facilitating a genuine understanding of one another's desires and preferences, as it unveils the hidden desires and fantasies that we all possess.

It enhances one's self-assurance when individuals can effectively express their desires and acquire them through proper articulation and inquiry.

It elicits sensations of arousal and stimulates both cerebral and emotional centers, targeting the intimate regions, mind, and core.

◆ ◆ ◆

Please engage in an imaginative approach rather than simply removing your clothing.

Your artistic ingenuity in articulating your sexual preferences, emotions, and desires, as well as in directing your partner's actions and words to enhance the overall sensual experience, appears limitless.

Occasionally, engaging in erotic dialogue can serve as a passionate expression of gratitude for the effort exerted in delivering pleasure.

Frequently, there arises a need to dictate the occurrence of an event that ignites one's ardor.

Occasionally, it is the mere whimsical depiction of a character or event that evokes an intense fervor when articulate

What will be my partner's reaction when I engage in provocative conversations during intimate moments?

It is highly probable that your romantic partner will express gratitude, possibly even through a gesture such as presenting flowers, for instigating a conversation that they have premeditated since the moment they acknowledged their feelings for you and desired emotional and physical closeness.

Many individuals find great allure in engaging in explicit discourse and intimate conversations; however, they often experience a degree of unease when attempting to initiate such dialogue.

Please be mindful that within a romantic relationship, all words hold significance, with the exception of those meant to cause harm. Fortunately, our communication is free from any intention to hurt one another.

Through the course of this voyage centered on individual expression, we are diligently rectifying the societal

limitations imposed upon language and communication, which restrict our ability to delve into and appreciate their vast possibilities. However, we can engage in activities that provide us with fulfillment, hence we proceed to embark on our initial seductive endeavors.

The intriguing aspect of sexting lies in its historical prevalence, as it existed long before being labeled 'sexting' in contemporary times, a term derived from the term 'texting'.

Present Times

While we have previously addressed the definition of sexting, let us now examine it once more. The definition of the word as provided by the Urban dictionary pertains to a suggestive message with the intention of establishing a romantic connection with the recipient at a later time. Nevertheless, not all instances of sexting are executed with the intention of engaging in sexual activity. It is a common practice to engage in teasing on a regular basis.

Netflexting

You might find yourself inquisitive about the nature of this. You are likely already acquainted with Netflix; however, if that is not the case, it is an online video

streaming platform that allows users to view films and television series on their computers and other electronic devices for a nominal monthly subscription fee. Profiles for every user can be found on this website. Netflexting entails strategically selecting movies or shows with titles that convey provocative themes or content with the purpose of conveying a specific thought or idea. They are included within the roster of another individual, thereby necessitating their elucidation of the titular communiqué.

In the past 5 to 10 years...
Sexting constituted predominantly as an exchange of verbal salutations accompanied by the presentation of a digital card. The card typically served as a professional business card, and the act of presenting the printed contact details was a symbolic representation of the request for a connection. Some individuals continue to employ this channel as a means to access the

contemporary form of sexting via electronic devices.

30 - Skywriting
Yes, skywriting. Although the messages were not suggestive, they conveyed such endearing sentiments that it is clear the man who commissioned the skywriter achieved his desired outcome. The majority of the skywritten messages comprised declarations of affection, along with requests for marriage.

Half a century ago: Vocal Communications Dispatch
Indeed, singing is a form of verbal communication. Nevertheless, it can be classified as a mode of sexting since it involves the transmission of a written message through the medium of singing to be delivered to the intended recipient. Indeed, considering the plethora of advanced technological devices available today, there is a compelling argument in favor of reviving singing telegrams as an effective means to inject greater

excitement or novelty into various situations.

A century in the past: The emergence of Morse Code.
Can you fathom receiving a 'request for a casual encounter' communicated through a sequence of electronic tones? Yes, this actually happened. In an era where telephones were unavailable, individuals who were deployed for military service desired means of communication, and this method became the preferred choice for fulfilling their need. \\\"Kiss me, STOP. I have a deep admiration for your physique, however, I must point out that it may lead to some misunderstanding.

Four Centuries Ago: Sonnets Transported via Avian Messengers
Certain individuals continue to employ sonnets penned in earlier times as a means of wooing contemporary women. In the past, this behavior was commonly regarded as a primary means of expressing romantic attachment,

commonly referred to as sexting. The gentleman would eloquently express the delightful flavor he imagined in the woman's lips, the captivating allure of her eyes, and the depth of his affection towards her. This conveyed a profoundly heartfelt sentiment, and indeed constituted a form of intimate electronic communication.

Observably, the practice of sexting has existed for as long as written or pictorial modes of communication have been present. Sexting entails the portrayal of intimate thoughts about another individual. Nevertheless, in contemporary times, the focus has shifted towards the crude element of physical closeness.

Chapter 4 – Patriarchal Supremacy

If you have not yet had the opportunity to peruse Fifty Shades of Grey, I must assert that you have yet to fully comprehend the passionate allure surrounding a woman's choice to

surrender complete authority over her sexual pursuits to a man. Men, possessing unchecked autonomy over their actions towards women, are capable of conjuring remarkable and explicit verbal expressions during passionate sexual encounters. Restraining her arms and securing them to the bed frame while uttering the words "My dear, you belong to me" can evoke a highly engaging dynamic between them. As he playfully explores her physique and tantalizingly delays her gratification, the experience can possess a tremendous allure.

Exploring her delicate areas through provocative speech and conduct

What if we were to utilize the vibrating device with her? I previously alluded to this, but it presents an exceptional opportunity for a couple to intimately connect on a profound level. If she appears to be eager for sexual activity, it would be advisable to delay gratification. Women typically appreciate it when men

assume control. As you discreetly retrieve the vibrator from beneath your pillow, you can firmly and gently hold her in position on the bed with her legs apart, directing the device towards those areas that crave greater stimulation, all while uttering the phrase "Let us proceed at a more measured pace, my dear; it is now time for pleasure." Naturally, once the vibrator begins to elicit visible reactions, there is no hindrance to her concurrently engaging with you in mutual pleasure. Make the right noises. Consider something more imaginative than the affirmative response of "yes," and you might pleasantly astonish one another.

The purpose of erotic communication is to entice, to tantalize, and to arouse one's partner in preparation for forthcoming activities. "Engage me fervently, my beloved!" might appear less tactful beyond intimate settings. However, if she devotes herself wholeheartedly to pleasuring you through a stimulating act of oral

intimacy, it would be appropriate to use a description of this nature. Alternatively, you could reposition her torso in a manner where your phallus is positioned between her chest, and politely request her to gently apply pressure to create a compressed effect." I would like to place myself between your breasts. I am certain she will accommodate. It is arousing and enjoyable. Allow her to engage in intimate activities with your genitals. If you are a female, allow him to engage in intimate contact with your breasts, genital area, and clitoral region. How is he expected to discern the appropriate stimuli to elicit your interest, if you fail to provide him with clear indications?

If you desire to gain insight into the thoughts of your partner during intimate moments, consider engaging her in conversation during such moments. Have her assume a position where she is positioned behind you, and kindly inquire about her experience or emotions. Inquiring whether you desire

additional quantity would not be deemed unreasonable. Under these circumstances, it would be quite appropriate to express that I am willing to provide you with all of my available resources. Experiment with various perspectives and engage in jovial conversation to discern the one that incites her the most.

In addition to employing profane language, there exist words of a less vulgar nature that men ought to bear in mind, ensuring the attainment of an appropriate equilibrium. Women should not be objectified as mere instruments for sexual gratification. While it is possible that they derive considerable pleasure from sexual activities, fundamentally, they are characterized as beings of emotional nature. If one reduces the act of sexual intercourse to vulgar language and mistreatment, it will not contribute to earning any form of favor or recognition. Certainly, it is acceptable to incorporate profane language and actively support her in

doing so. However, it is important to bear in mind that women also require emotional care and that a harmonious blend of both elements is crucial for sustaining a thriving and engaging relationship.

It is important to acknowledge that engaging in sexual intimacy involves the active participation of both partners. By creating an atmosphere of mutual encouragement and effective communication in the bedroom, one can achieve the desired balance. For instance, there is no inherent issue with positioning her on her stomach while securely fastening her to the headboard, subsequently cradling her breasts and affirming, "You possess the most exceptional bosom!", as it effectively boosts her self-assurance. An alternative approach would be to restrain her hands to the bedhead, positioning her in a way that allows you to maintain complete dominance, engaging in intimate contact from a posterior position and verbalizing your sensations upon

penetration. That sensation is quite pleasurable, my love. Let us engage in an intimate encounter enhanced by the use of vaginal creams, providing potentially heightened sexual satisfaction.

The predicament lies in the fact that individuals are not adequately educated about the mechanics of sexual intercourse. It becomes necessary to engage in experimentation within the confines of a mutually understanding and familiar partnership, in order to discern one's boundaries and limitations. Engaging in spontaneous moments, such as removing one's undergarments, can serve as a powerful source of arousal. Take advantage of a suitable moment, such as when you find yourselves alone in the residence, to broach the subject of her removing her undergarments, particularly after having enjoyed a delightful meal prepared by her. Addressing her with affectionate words and expressing a desire to sensually explore her body in a downwards direction may potentially

ignite her arousal. Women love getting attention.

If you find her extremely attractive, why not express your affection by removing her undergarments and articulating your desire to engage in an intimate encounter, whilst acknowledging that she has a captivating effect on your emotions. Following a formal dinner event, prior to clearing the table, engage in intimate activity upon its surface while engaging in risqué conversation, treating your partner as if she were your professional secretary. "Well, Miss .... What did I mention about the consequences that would ensue if your behavior were unsatisfactory? Let's make it a lighthearted conversation. Create something profoundly surprising, if you so desire, however, ensure her full knowledge and consent, and let her enthusiasm be equal to your own. That is the point at which it truly becomes excellent.

Employing vulgar language to demonstrate the intentions and plans you possess for her

If she exhibits a tolerance for the usage of profanity, then it is reasonably permissible for you to employ it, but remain attentive. A woman who is your committed companion desires a deeper connection than being merely objectified or sexualized. However, in situations where you have shared experiences with erotic literature or similar prompting, there may be rare occasions where the use of such language can be impactful. "You will undoubtedly repent your actions," you may counter her initiation and subsequently assume control, allowing her to witness the seriousness of your intentions.

Sex is a remarkable experience. It is not limited to activities conducted in darkness with the absence of light. Please illuminate the room and scrutinize her physique in a manner that conveys your profound admiration.

Caress her skin, gently touch and inquire whether she finds it pleasurable. Inquire about her personal aspirations and endeavor to satisfy them while aiming for reciprocity in fulfilling your own desires. Effective communication is an essential component of a satisfying sexual experience. It encompasses more than mere vocal expressions and reaching a peak of pleasure. If you hold the belief that this is the sole essence of intimate encounters, then it is imperative that you acquire the skills to employ verbal communication to foster a mutually fulfilling sexual connection with your partner.

The earlier you take action, the earlier you can indulge in pleasurable intimacy, extending beyond the confines of the bedroom. Arrange the bathtub decoratively, partake in a shower together, or engage in intimate activity in the presence of an open hearth. Quietly utter explicit language into her auditory organ and actively motivate her to reciprocate in kind. If it leads to the

restoration of your sexual well-being, then it merits the effort.

Expressing a desire to fully immerse myself in your intimate core is a highly arousing statement to share, moments before providing you with an unparalleled experience of oral pleasure. It pertains to adhering to propriety. It is not imperative that you exercise caution in expressing yourself. It signifies that you must possess a profound understanding of her character, allowing you to anticipate the amorous attraction she will develop towards you in response to your words. If you are uncertain, consider engaging in an extended period of intimate prelude throughout the entire evening.

The issue lies in our tendency to overlook the profound sense of intimacy inherent in the act of engaging in sexual intercourse. People engage in intimate activities as though it is a prescribed responsibility or a mandated duty. Commence verbal communication –

initiate the articulation of your emotions. Articulate your thoughts without hesitation or reluctance, ensuring that there is a mutual understanding and alignment between both parties. Once you reach that point, it becomes quite impressive and you are capable of achieving remarkable feats in collaboration. Adopt mutually alluring pseudonyms or incorporate them into your intimate discourse. If she possesses exquisitely developed breasts, for instance, kindly express your appreciation. If he possesses the physique of a male deer, please relay this information to him. Contemplate alternate monikers that effectively convey the intended meaning between one another.

Engaging in explicit conversation involves complete transparency and sharing without any reservations with your significant other. Indeed, it is natural that there will be occasions when one experiences a lack of inclination towards engaging in sexual

activities. That is also acceptable and should not significantly affect your sexual life unless it occurs with excessive frequency. If such a situation arises, it is imperative to engage in a dialogue that aims to effectively redress any concerns or issues that you may possess.

Nicholas

SHIT. Bennett, my closest companion, who held the role of pack beta in our collective, was present at my place of residence. He was attending to the repair of my lawn mower. That would typically not pose an issue.

However, I was accompanied by Avan.

I inadvertently left the engine of the truck running, thereby inadvertently securing Avan's presence within. My truck was equipped with a mechanism that ensured the doors remained locked from the inside. "Stay here. I'll be right back."

I hastily entered the garage, where Bennet was enveloped by an array of components. "I would like to engage in a conversation with you," I conveyed.

He used a cloth to clean his hands. "What did you do? I am eagerly anticipating listening to this."

"Kindly refrain from further vocalization," I expressed, acknowledging the undue level of assertiveness in my communication.

His eyebrows shot up. What is the root cause of your current state of stress?

I endeavored to compose myself. "I witnessed an incident wherein a hiker fell victim to an assault by a group of coyotes," I mentioned.

"And?" he asked.

I endeavored to elucidate all aspects, however, prior to broaching the notion of Avan's potential status as an omega, a cacophonous fracture interrupted my discourse.

Fuck. Avan had gotten out.

Bennett whirled around. "What was that?"

"Oh no." I hurriedly made my way to the window. He is disembarking from the vehicle.

"What on earth is transpiring?" Bennet exclaimed with exasperation.

I swiftly exited the premises, taking a momentary pause to observe my vehicle,

noting the shattered window and the door agape. Then I kept running.

Bennett pursued me while vociferating, yet I was unable to cast a glance in his direction.

We swiftly descended along the surfaced section of the driveway and proceeded onto the gravel pathway.

I discerned a distant sound. It appeared to be the sound of muted cries. Was that my mate? Bennett hastened towards me and seized hold of my arm.

"May I inquire if there is anyone present nearby?" he inquired.

"That is precisely the topic that I am attempting to address with you," I retorted with urgency.

He sniffed the air. "What's that smell?"

I emitted a deep growl from within as the alluring aroma reached my nostrils.

The aroma emanated strongly from an omega on the verge of entering their heat cycle.

My omega.

Dammit. Avan's innate instincts were likely stimulated in my presence. They

had been in a state of dormancy, but that state had ceased.

I asserted ownership, articulating my dominance by revealing my teeth to my acquaintance.

Startled, he retreated, raising his hands. "What's going on?"

Ugh. I was expressing my dissatisfaction towards my closest acquaintance, who also held the role of my subordinate. I trusted him completely. I needed to pull myself together.

Once more, I was abruptly overwhelmed by the most exquisite scent I had ever encountered. I inhaled through my oral cavity while making concerted effort to concentrate.

"Holy shit," Bennett said. "He's an omega, right? Hence, the reason behind your current state of distress. That is the reason for your strong sense of territoriality.

His fragrance bore a resemblance to the harmonious amalgamation of sugar and honey. It was unlike any experience I had previously come across.

Did Bennet inquire about his state of arousal?

I exhaled. "I kindly request that you remain in your current location," I relayed. "He doesn't know."

"Are you declining my assistance?" he inquired.

Negative, I have no intention of engaging in any form of aggression towards you.

"Okay," he said. "I'll go home. However, please do not hesitate to inform me if you require my assistance."

I embraced him firmly, clutching tightly onto his figure. "Thank you.

I resumed running hastily.

Currently, Avan had approached an oak tree and commenced ascending its lower branches. I was unable to tolerate observing his attempts to flee, and I adamantly refused to let any harm befall him due to potential falls. I experienced an innate inclination to provide him with the assurance that I would not cause him any harm. Avan, please desist! I merely seek to engage in conversation.

I successfully arrived at the foundation of the tree.

He cast a disapproving gaze upon me from a vantage point midway above.

He was exhibiting signs of heightened sexual arousal, and despite this, he maintained a persistent glare and continued to display resistance towards me - his chosen partner. I greatly appreciated that he did not yield easily in his stance.

I raised my hands. Rest assured, I pose no harm to you. I simply desire to engage in conversation. I am aware that you may have inquiries." "I understand that you might have queries." "I acknowledge the presence of questions on your part." "I recognize the possibility of you having concerns."

"Right. Hence, you are pursuing me across an expanse of land. As you desire a conversation. And the only actions you have taken involve deception. What is the basis for me to place trust in any of your statements?"

I sighed. "You're right."

Could you kindly provide an explanation of the current situation?

"I will. If you would be so kind as to descend."

"No," he insisted.

An electric surge coursed through my veins. God, he was hot.

He cast a piercing gaze in my direction. His deep, auburn eyes gleamed in the twilight of the fading afternoon.

The frisson grew stronger. I refrained from physical contact with him, yet mere proximity elicited a strong impulse within me to declare my unwavering loyalty to him. This form of loyalty was an inherent aspect of forming a bond with a partner, particularly in the case of assuming the role of an Alpha. Had I approached this matter in a different manner, things might have been better.

I am determined to persuade him, regardless of the challenges. Despite the potential discontent that it might cause among my group. Despite the eventuality of his departure from the group.

STRATEGIES FOR ENGAGING CHILDREN AGED 9 TO 12 IN DISCOURSE REGARDING SEXUALITY

It is imperative that you commence addressing issues of sexism and sexualization at this stage of development. To initiate dialogues, one could make references to media examples or local anecdotes, such as an elderly woman who holds the belief that males ought to maintain short hair.

While these discussions may elicit distressing emotions, they serve to foster resilience in children and provide compelling narratives of individuals who have triumphed over societal biases. Additionally, highlight the progress achieved, notably the rise in the representation of women in STEM careers.

In the midst of this stage characterized by emotional and social transformation, it is especially common for girls to encounter challenges pertaining to their

self-perception regarding their physical appearance. It is imperative for parents to consistently inquire about the emotions and curiosities of their children.

It essentially involves consistently emphasizing the natural phenomenon of bodily changes that occur during this particular stage of development.

Promoting sexual health and wellness should be an additional objective to pursue universally. It is advisable to initiate discussions about sexual preferences and safer sexual practices at approximately 11 years of age. This concept is somewhat disconcerting, yet it holds significant importance as empirical evidence indicates that children exhibit enhanced decision-making abilities when they possess an understanding of potential hazards. You are advised to emphasize a range of contraceptive methods and provide a rudimentary explanation of their mechanisms.

It is advisable to engage in periodic conversations regarding internet safety and further enhance the existing digital norms and principles, as individuals within this demographic frequently enjoy increased online autonomy. For instance, engage in a candid dialogue to determine the potential illegality of disseminating photographs depicting oneself or others unclothed or engaging in explicit sexual acts. They may face allegations of engaging in the production or distribution of child pornography.

Inquire of your child about their understanding of the concept of "exhibiting respectful behavior on social media." Furthermore, leverage prominent news events such as instances of sexting or online bullying as a catalyst to initiate discussions with your child regarding their anticipated reactions in similar situations.

How to broach the topic of sexual education with your adolescent

When your children reach the stage of adolescence, initiating an early discussion about sex and sexuality truly yields significant benefits. Provided that you have exhibited a willingness to engage in discussions pertaining to those subjects. It is highly likely that your children will experience increased comfort in engaging in conversation and seeking clarification from you.

Nevertheless, if you have refrained from engaging in discussions regarding sexuality with your adolescent thus far, I strongly recommend arranging a dedicated time for such a conversation and explicitly stating your intent to do so. For the majority of children, the mere act of hearing those words proves to be highly reassuring.

While it is generally advisable to reduce the frequency of lecturing, it is of utmost importance to provide adolescents with accurate information regarding contraception. It would be advisable to

consider the provision of condoms or the arrangement of a medical consultation for the purpose of administering chemical birth control.

It is imperative to consistently address the topic of consent within the context of sexual relationships. Take into account strategies to support them in resisting peer influence and addressing issues of relationship violence.
The matter of drugs and alcohol and their potential impact on judgment should be addressed concurrently with these subjects.

It is essential to engage in frequent discussions regarding harmonious partnerships. I recommend discussing school acquaintances if your child exhibits hesitance in disclosing personal information about themselves. You may also wish to explore previous encounters with romantic partnerships.

Ultimately, concerning adolescents, it is desirable to grant your offspring the

freedom to evaluate potential hazards and arrive at prudent conclusions. Sex education places significant emphasis on imparting the knowledge that young individuals possess an innate intuition and instinct, which they are both capable and obligated to heed. You are cultivating your child's readiness to achieve this goal by addressing the relevant topics in a timely manner.